ACT FAST, SAVE LIVES
An Illustrated Stroke Survival Guide

Mary Karol, Author

2020 © Survive a Stroke Foundation

Dedication Page

To Rose, who wanted to live – but didn't get help. A room full of RNs didn't recognize she was having a stroke.
This booklet is for all the readers who want to live after a medical emergency such as a stroke. Learn as you age how to prepare for any kind of medical emergency.
For more information, read Broken Trust, A Stroke Survival Guide, Every Minute Counts; and Aging in America, A Cautionary Tale of Wrongful Death in Elder Care

About the Author

The author, Mary Karol, is a former graduate law school professor, a frequent speaker for continuing education, and published in numerous business journals. She is active in estate planning and elder law organizations. Donations from this booklet go to the Survive a Stroke Foundation.

Strokes are Sneaky You Don't Know When They Will Appear

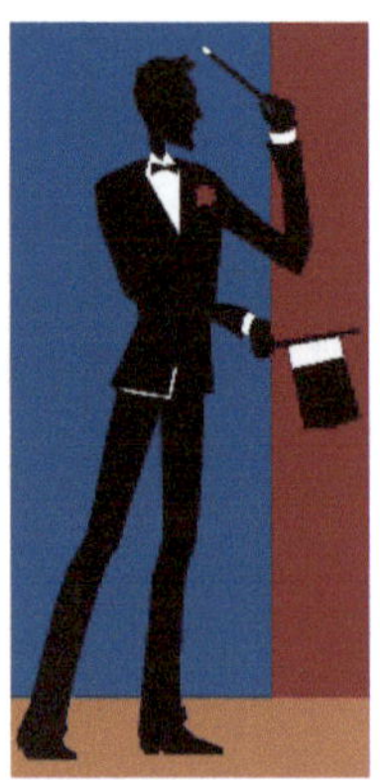

Table of Contents

5

Introduction

This easy to read and understand illustrated booklet will help you, or someone you love, survive a stroke and other medical emergencies. Why is this critical to learn today? Medical emergencies can happen at any time. You don't get a second chance very often to recognize and respond to a stroke. It is an example of a medical emergency that is common as people age, and may now even occur with younger persons.

In 2020 it was discovered that even though typically considered a lung infection, COVID-19 has been found to cause blood clots that can lead to severe stroke. Experts say that this can happen in any patient regardless of age, and even in those with few or no symptoms.

This booklet is based on a true story. It can happen to anyone unable to help themselves in a medical emergency. You cannot count on the health care system to help you. Read on and you will understand why the trust in that system is broken.

Everyone should recognize the signs of a stroke. Any of the stroke symptoms in Part One is a reason to call 911. Don't rely on others to diagnose what is and is not a stroke in progress. Do not rely on anyone. Protect those you love yourself in any medical emergency.

Part One

Pictures Tell the Story of a Stroke: Lessons to be Learned Now, While There is Time

What are the warning signs that a stroke has started?

Look over the illustrations below and remember them. If any of these happen, you should be put on notice and ready to call 911 immediately!!

Look at each of the following examples and do not ignore any of them if they happen. Any one of these can be the signal of a stroke. Many think that a stroke has to have a droopy face. That is not true. Do not wait for someone else to make the decision that something is wrong. No matter where you are, others may make a mistake and do nothing. Do not hesitate to act and do not be embarrassed. You are recognizing an emergency!
If you don't act, the consequences are often death or disability for you or the ones you love.

#1
Sudden Event or Change ?

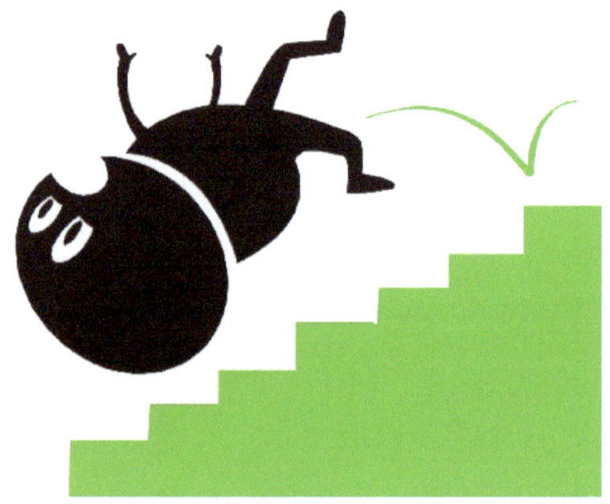

You, or someone you are with, all of a sudden undergoes a sudden unexplained change ? This can be a stroke !

#2
Confused ?

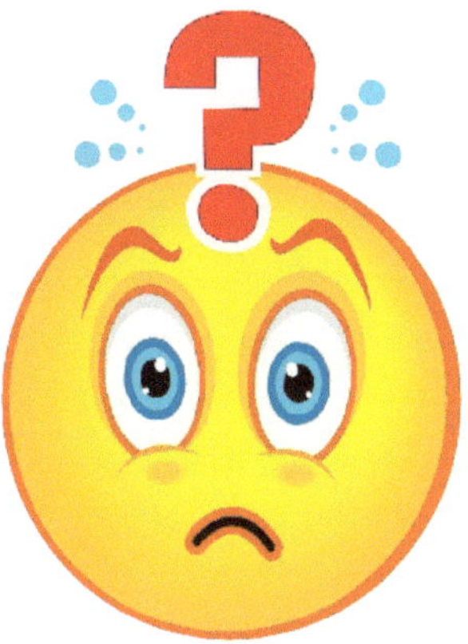

You, or someone you are with, all of a sudden becomes confused ? This can be a stroke !

#3
Headache ?

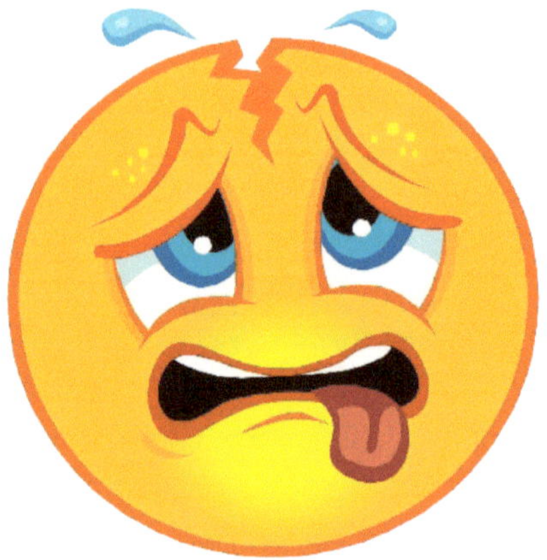

You, or someone you are with, all of a sudden has a terrible headache ? This can be a stroke !

#4
Trouble Speaking or Not Speaking ?

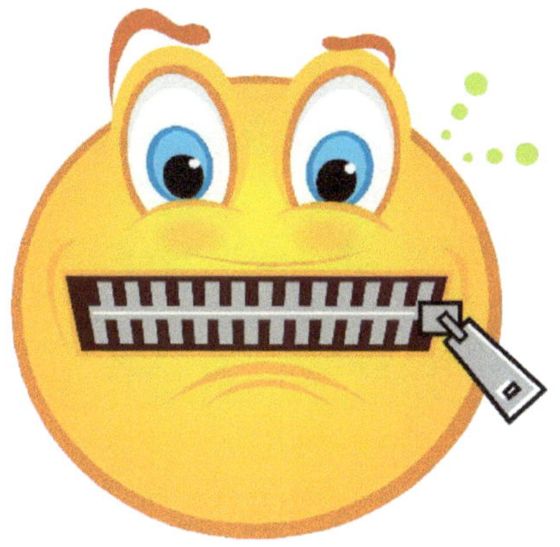

You, or someone you are with, all of a sudden has trouble talking or isn't talking at all ? This can be a stroke !

#5
Cannot Swallow Easily ?

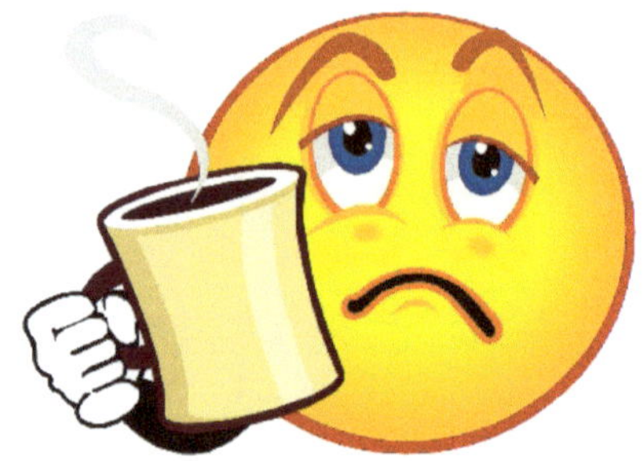

You, or someone you are with, all of a sudden has trouble swallowing their pills, drink or food ? This can be a stroke !

#6
Paralyzed or Droopy ?

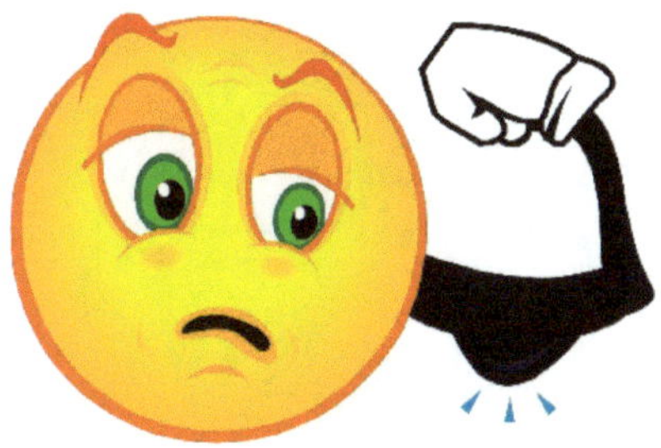

You, or someone you are with, all of a sudden has an arm, leg or side of the face become droopy or paralyzed ? This can be a stroke !

Any of those six examples can signal a stroke and the clock starts ticking

Time to Act Fast – Every Minute Counts

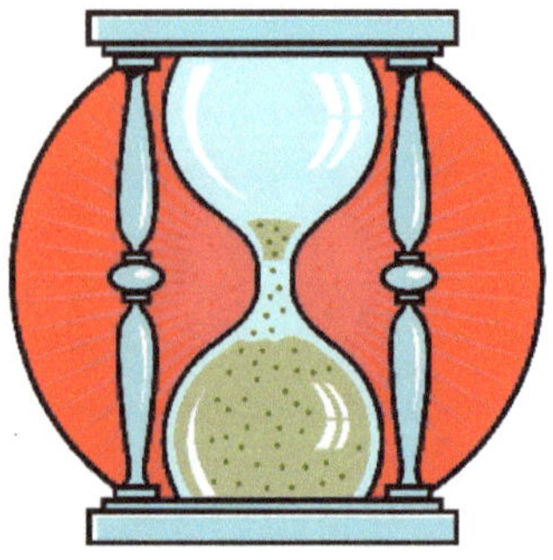

Telephone Right Away
Call 911!

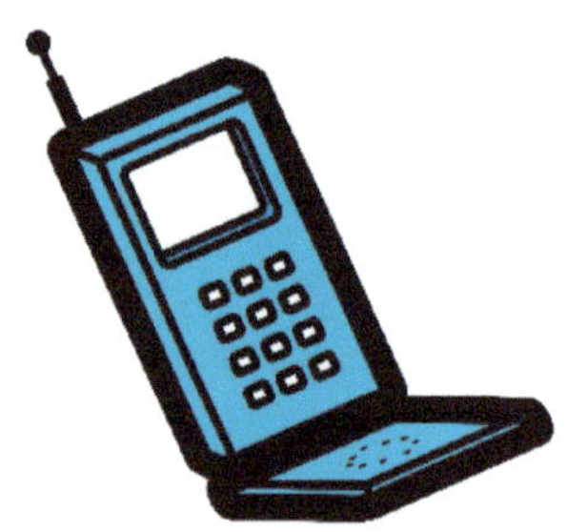

Get An Ambulance to the Nearest Hospital

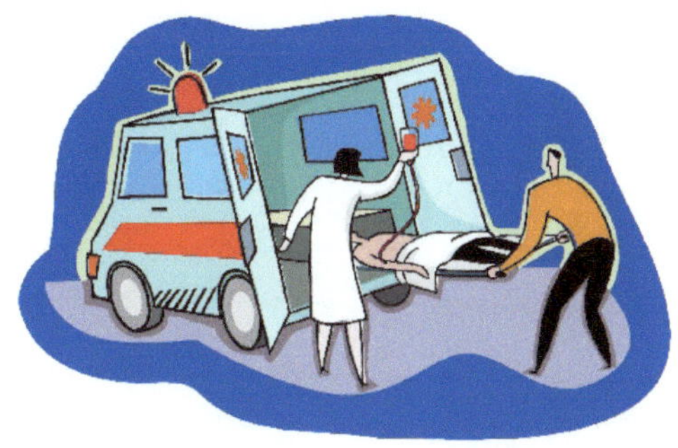

Get to a hospital emergency room (ER) in an ambulance. Do not drive to the ER.

A stroke is an emergency and will be given the highest priority by the emergency room at the hospital when an ambulance brings you. The emergency response team in an ambulance will call in to the ER that they may have a stroke victim, so the ER is prepared to act when you arrive.

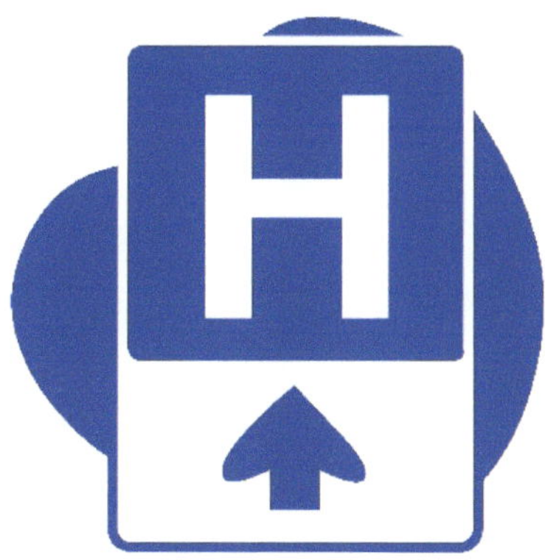

In the Emergency Room the doctors can determine if it's a stroke and if there is a blood clot or if it's bleeding in the brain.

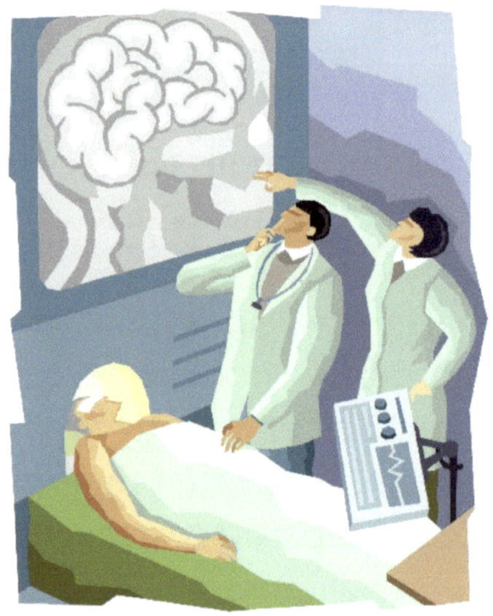

A drug can be injected within 3-4 hours after a stroke if there is a clot to break up the clot. The brain starts to die every minute that it is deprived of blood flow for oxygen. And, if you cannot make that 3-4 hour window, there still is time.

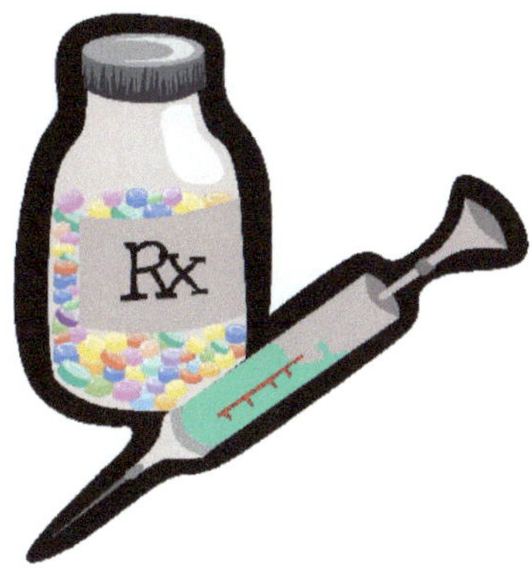

Don't let that precious window of time pass. Up to 8 hours after the onset of a stroke, there are still procedures that can save a life !

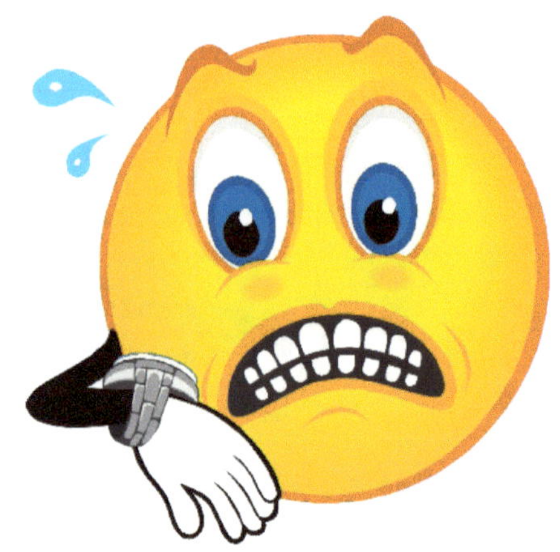

If needed, the hospital ER will have you airlifted to a hospital that is certified as an acute primary stroke center after you are stabalized. Primary stroke centers are prepared to treat acute stroke victims.

Don't end up with a broken heart because no one called 911 in time. Don't rely on the decisions or actions of others – they can be wrong.

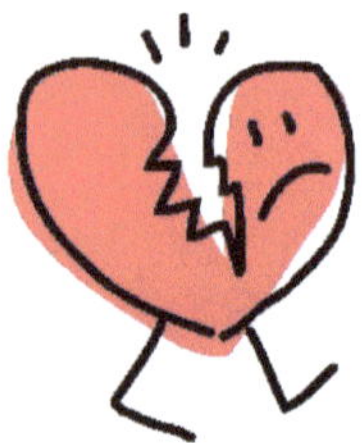

Don't say good bye to the ones you love because no one called 911.

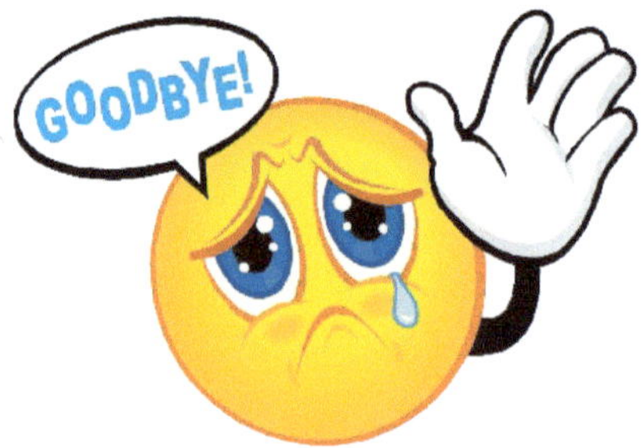

There is no reason for a person to die from a stroke who could have been saved. If it is someone you love, its very painful.

Stroke is one of the leading causes of death in the United States. It has been linked in 2020 to COVID-19 for persons of all ages.

A stroke not recognized and treated properly, if it doesn't cause a death, may cause a serious disability. **Stroke is a leading cause of disability in the United States. It can put you in a nursing home for years.**

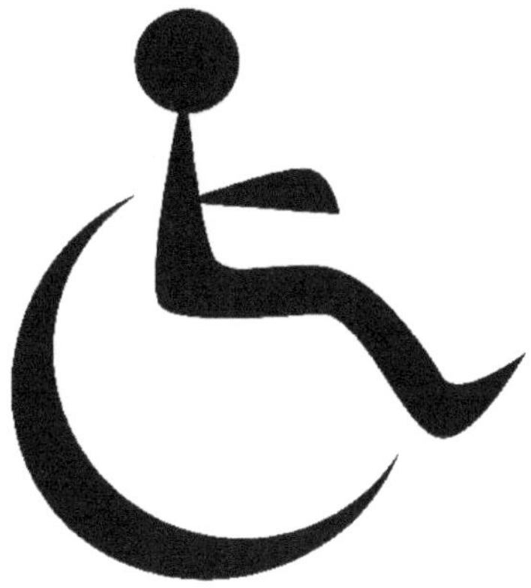

Don't Let this Happen To You or To Someone You Love.

Part Two

Quiz for Anyone at Any Age

#1. Someone was fine the last time you saw them, and then all of a sudden they are not acting right. Do you call 911 to be sure they are OK or wait?

#2. All the nurses in a health care facility say the person is sick with an infection, and it's not a stroke, this is all of a sudden. Do you call 911 to be sure the nurses are right?

#3. Someone drools out their food or beverage. Do you call 911 to be sure they are OK?

#4. Does someone always have a droopy face when they are having a stroke?

#5. You suspect someone is having a stroke, do you ask others what they think or do you call 911?

#6. If you call 911 and it turns out the person is not having a stroke, are you in trouble?

#7. Do only "old" people have strokes?

#8. If a person has had a temporary stroke before, or has atrial fibrillation (heart) – is there a good chance a sudden change is a stroke?

#9. At the ER, if you think there might be any chance the person is having stroke, should you insist on a brain scan?

#10. Can a person having a stroke ask you to call 911?

If you have any doubt if it might be a stroke,
will you call 911?

Answers

If you think the quiz was too easy – don't laugh.
Never take a chance if it is a stroke.
Always call 911.

Practice the quiz questions with family and friends
And in any health care community or residence where you or your
loved ones may reside

#1, #2 and #3 Yes

#4, #5 and #6 No
Always call 911

#7 People any age can have a stroke

#8 Yes
These are precursors to a later stroke
BEWARE!

#9 Yes
If in the ER, don't be turned away
Demand the most care

#10 No
A person having a stroke usually cannot ask for help
You must help them by calling 911

Always error on the side of caution and call 911

Part Three

Important Documents

Do you have these documents and are they current?

Out of date documents will not help you in a medical emergency

Out of date documents may contribute to your death

If you don't know what these documents are- please find out today

Living will

DNR Order – Do Not Resuscitate Order

Durable Power of Attorney for Health Care

POLST (Physicians Order for Life Sustaining Treatment)

See next page for brief summary definitions

REMEMBER, A STROKE IS SURVIVEABLE

THERE IS LIFE AFTER A STROKE

A **Living Will** is a legal document where the person designates if they want life support continued if they are incapacitated and in a "terminal condition", an "end stage condition", or **in a** "persistent vegetative state". A living will may also be known as a personal directive, physician's directive, or medical directive, depending upon the State where the person lives.

A Durable power of attorney for health care/Medical power of attorney or is a legal document where the person gives another person the power to make health care decisions for them if they are unable. In may also be called a Designation of Health Care Surrogate, Health Care Proxy, or similar names depending upon the State where the person lives.

If you have both a living will type of document and a health care power of attorney, some states combine them into one document. These legal documents are known as advance directives.

A **DNR** is a document that specifies that the person does not want to be resuscitated. When you are admitted to the hospital you may be asked what you would like medical personnel to do in the event that your heart stops working.

Be careful if you choose this and you later have a medical emergency that is not about your heart. Medical care providers may look to the DNR and decide you do not want to live!

All persons should have these legal documents, called advance care directives, which outline your desires related to end-of-life care in the event you cannot speak for yourself. In addition, ask your primary care provider to explain and perhaps fill out with you a POLST, Physician Orders for Life-Sustaining Treatment, form, which is a medical order (one copy is for you to keep, and one goes in your medical record) that outlines the treatment and interventions you are okay with in a medical emergency. (Different states vary the POLST program – you should check online) A nursing home or residential care facility may force you to sign this type of document and may not keep it updated thereafter.

If you are admitted to the hospital and are not asked your preferences for life-sustaining treatment, you must let the doctor treating you know your wishes.

Every time you go in or out of a medical facility such as a hospital to a nursing home and back, the POLST type of document must be updated.

POLST is **a medical** order that gives seriously ill patients more control over their care. A **POLST** form is neither an **advance directive** nor a replacement for **advance directives**. However, both **advance directives** and **POLST** forms are helpful documents for communicating patient wishes when appropriately used. **The most recent document will control.**

A POLST BECOMES A LIFE OR DEATH DOCUMENT IN A MEDICAL EMERGENCY SUCH AS A STROKE – SO MAKE SURE A POLST IS CURRENT TO THE VERY DAY IF THERE IS A MEDICAL EMERGENCY

POLST orders are also known by other names in some states: Medical Orders for Life-Sustaining Treatment (**MOLST**), Medical Orders on Scope of Treatment (MOST), Physician's Orders on Scope of Treatment (POST) or Transportable Physician Orders for Patient Preferences (TPOPP).

Disclaimer

This booklet is presented for educational purposes only. Under no circumstances should it be mistaken for professional legal or medical advice, nor is it at all intended to be taken as such. The commentary and other contents simply reflect the opinion of the author alone.

www.ingramcontent.com/pod-product-compliance
Lightning Source LLC
Chambersburg PA
CBHW040933110726
48006CB00001B/172